THE DOCTORS' SECRETS

SECRETS

to a Lifetime of Clear Skin

The easy-to-read, easy-to-use
guide to stopping acne.

———

Katie Rodan, M.D., and Kathy Fields, M.D.

Introduction

While it may not be fair, it has always been true: We are judged by our appearance. And problem skin can profoundly affect the quality of your life.

At first, you might not believe that something so common—and biologically ordinary—as acne could have life-changing consequences, but it can. As doctors, we know that acne affects all aspects of a person's life—from school success and work performance, to personal relationships and self-esteem.

We see firsthand the heartache acne causes in our patients, and we've experienced that heartache ourselves. Truth be told, it was our own struggles with acne that motivated us to create an at-home treatment focused on both healing and helping to prevent breakouts. Our innovative approach has been revolutionary, making the Proactiv® product the number-one acne-treatment system in America.

In your fight against acne, knowledge is a key weapon. So, on the pages that follow, we share 30 "secrets" taken straight from our dermatology practices. We also offer a new program—called Proactiv365™—that is available to you, as a current Proactiv® customer, for no additional charge.

Proactiv365™ program includes online diagnostics and a comprehensive database of helpful information in an easily searchable Q&A format. Most importantly, you enjoy around-the-clock access to an expert team of Skin Care Advisors—trained by us—for personal one-on-one guidance to help you achieve and maintain a clear complexion.

As dermatologists, we understand that everyone's skin is different. Your experience with Proactiv® will be unique. So, whenever you have questions or concerns, professional help is standing by and included as part of your experience with Proactiv®.

We care about your success. Our goal is to see you enjoy all the happiness that a clear, healthy-looking complexion can bring!

With best wishes,

Katie Rodan, M.D., and Kathy Fields, M.D.
Board-Certified Dermatologists
Co-Creators of Proactiv Acne Treatment System

1
Acne thrives on your indecision.

Acne. Pimples. Breakouts. Blemishes.
Blackheads. Whiteheads. Papules. Pustules.
Zits. Spots.

Too many names for something you hate to talk about but can't stop thinking about.

All the time. Once a month.

When you're stressed. Or not.

When eating the wrong stuff. Or eating anything.

You skip the snapshot. You just want freedom from your acne.

So now is the time to decide that you are going to do what it takes to get acne out of your life for good.

Decide, commit, never look back.

There is a path to a life without acne, and this book will help you get there. Today is Day One.

2

Acne is everywhere and it never, ever gives up.

Acne itself—formally (and appropriately) known as *acne vulgaris*—is defined medically as everything from blackheads to full-on, all-over-your-face breakouts.

Think those little whiteheads or once-a-month "undergrounders" aren't acne? Think again.

Acne is the number-one skin disease in the world. It doesn't discriminate based on race, ethnicity, age, gender … it is an equal opportunity offender. In the United States, some 85% of us have it at one time or another—and not just before proms.

Even the lucky clear-skinned teens often develop acne as adults.

And once your skin starts breaking out, you learn that acne is relentless. It is the gift that keeps on giving. So don't wait to "outgrow" acne, because it could be years.

Or never.

Acne never gives up, so neither can you.

3

Acne is common, complex, chronic and NOT curable. But it IS controllable.

You now know how common acne is—millions and millions of people have it.

But you need to know what you are up against.

Acne is complex. It offers no easy way out.

Acne is chronic, too—which, in doctors' lingo, means it can last a very long time: 5–7 years in a teen or decades in an adult.

We hate to break the news, but acne also is not curable—not by prescription pills, not by the best topicals.

The good news is that, with the right combination of medicines, those with acne can enjoy skin that's as clear and healthy-looking as someone who has no acne at all. The secret is finding the right combination of medicines and skin-care treatments that work for you.

4

"First, we make our habits. Then, our habits make us."

The great thing about habits is that good ones are just as hard to break as bad ones.

You brush your teeth twice a day, right? That's a great example of a good habit—proactive and preventive self-care for teeth.

Now is the time for you to acquire a clear-skin habit.

Once your skin is blemish free—and it will be—stick to your daily maintenance routine.

Why?

Your skin is clear because your medicines are working, not because your acne has been cured.

Stop your acne routine and blemishes may very well revisit your face within a month or two.

Clearing ends the first stage of your journey. It is not the beginning of the end; it is the end of the beginning.

5

Acne is not your fault. There's lots of blame to go around.

Chocolate, french fries and a soda or occasionally forgetting to wash off your makeup do not cause acne.

These are factors that may bring on a flare-up, but they are not the root cause of your acne.

In other words, acne is not your fault.

Your heredity and your hormones are to blame.

That doesn't mean there aren't things you can do to help. Perhaps the biggest acne trigger is STRESS. The more stress you have, the more your body releases the "fight or flight" hormone, cortisol, which can make your acne worse, which causes even more anxiety, which further increases stress, which—well, you get the picture.

So cutting out sweets and drinking pure rainwater and doing a lot of things you've probably already tried won't make a difference.

6

Turns out, you *are* what you eat ... sometimes.

So it's a "myth" that chocolate makes you break out.

Here's a big "but": While diet isn't the cause of acne, it turns out that in some people certain foods can trigger the acne process, resulting in a worsening of your breakout.

The main culprits reported include iodine (which is added to salt and found in fish); the hormones present in meat and milk; and high-glycemic foods, also known as "junk foods."

So if you think certain foods are your face's foe, keep a daily diary of everything you eat, and look for a link between your diet and an acne flare-up a couple of weeks later. If you pinpoint the culprit, common sense says it would be better to avoid it than to eat it.

7

The sun is acne's friend—not your skin's.

One of the oddest myths about acne is that the sun is a key ally in your fight—particularly in drying pimples.

If by "good for acne" we mean "it encourages more acne," then, yes, the sun is good for acne.

Let's be clear: Sun exposure makes acne much worse and should be avoided.

A tan can temporarily hide a red, broken-out complexion.

But where did that get you?

As that tan fades, your skin starts to shed more cells—which clog pores and trigger more breakouts a few weeks down the road.

Keep in mind that some good deeds will not go unpunished. Some sunscreens can also make acne worse. To prevent pores from clogging, look for "non-comedogenic," "non-acnegenic" or "oil-free" on the sunscreen product package or label.

8

Even when your days of acne are behind you, wear sun protection.

Whoever coined the term "healthy tan" was totally uninformed.

Acne aside, the sun's rays have a bunch of bad consequences for your skin—acute burns, cancers, pigmented spots, wrinkles, premature aging, permanent widening of the pores and dilated blood vessels.

From sunup to sundown, 365 days a year—every day is "sunday."

Sun damage is cumulative and small exposures really add up.

There are two kinds of ultraviolet sunlight: UVB "burning" rays are the ones that, well, cause a sunburn. However, the majority of the UV damage comes from the UVA "aging" rays. These are the insidious ones.

Wear only "broad spectrum" sunscreen—which means it blocks both wavelengths. Look for zinc oxide, avobenzone or Mexoryl™ on the "active ingredient" list.

9

First, do no harm.

That sage advice to physicians is very apt for self-care.

We hesitate to call to your attention the bizarre array of home remedies for acne—lest you be tempted—but please do not try to clear your skin with antifungal cream, dishwashing liquid, lemon juice, hemorrhoid cream (what?), toothpaste, baking soda, egg whites, milk of magnesia, garlic, newborn baby urine (ineffective and not as easy to get as you might think), corn starch, hydrogen peroxide, garden mud, vinegar or window cleaner.

Don't let desperation take you down a path to nowhere, or worse—wasting valuable time and money.

10

The one thing you must NEVER do is sometimes what you most WANT to do.

In life, there are plenty of "rules" telling us what we can and cannot do. In the acne world, the big No-No is popping zits.

The temptation to pop must be resisted with all your strength because, while gratifying at one level, it has terrible—and sometimes permanent—consequences.

First, it drives bacteria deeper, setting up everything for a worse infection to come. Second, you can damage the surrounding skin tissue, which can cause scars that mark you for life.

What to do instead? Apply an ice cube to reduce inflammation. Then follow with a medicated spot treatment—something with benzoyl peroxide, sulfur or salicylic acid to speed healing. A little concealer—yes, even for the guys—and you're on your way today with the assurance that you will also have a clear tomorrow.

Later, crater.

11

If there are to be permanent marks on our skin, let them be voluntary.

While tattoos are something we generally advise against, at least many of those with "ink" knew what they were doing when they decided to permanently mark their skin.

But an acne scar? Some say scars are souvenirs, but who wants a permanent reminder of this nightmare?

Unfortunately, scars are a real possibility—especially if acne is left untreated.

With today's medicines for clearing and preventing breakouts, no one should have acne scars anymore.

The longer you live with your breakouts, the greater the risk of permanent scarring.

Depending upon the severity of inflammation, even a short-term case of acne can cause long-term scarring.

And don't confuse scars with discoloration. Those dark spots after a blemish are called "post-inflammatory hyperpigmentation." These marks are not permanent, but may take weeks to heal.

12

You can't even GIVE acne away.

Sometimes your acne can make you feel like an outcast.

However, you'll be rid of it soon, so it's good for your future "clear self" to know that acne is absolutely not contagious.

No one can catch acne.

The *P. acnes* bacteria that cause acne colonize everybody's face—even that of your friend with the perfect complexion.

The process of how those bacteria cause breakouts depends on many other individual factors—including the type of oil your glands make and how easily your pores clog.

Sharing pillowcases or dancing cheek to cheek with someone experiencing a full-on breakout will not make your acne worse.

So don't shy away. Acne is already a lonely experience.

13

Apply to affected areas only—NOT.

We are probably the last two people to tell you to *not* follow directions, but "spot" treating pimples by applying medicines to "affected areas only" is a game that your acne wants you to play—it flourishes while you're playing catch-up.

Why?

Because that red zit is actually the very *last* stage in the acne process. By the time a pimple erupts, you're witnessing the *finale,* not the beginning.

Full-face acne treatments are about shoring up the dams; spot treatments are clean-ups after the flood.

In a very literal way, the big red "spot" you're treating today is SOOOO two weeks ago!

Using a *daily,* medicated system for your whole face is the way to help prevent pimples at the source (i.e., deep inside your pores).

And those are directions you *should* follow.

14
A pimple is not simple.

Why does it take two or three weeks to make a pimple? Because acne is complicated!

The first thing to know is that every day your skin sheds lots of dead cells.

How many? Try one million dead skin cells every 40 minutes.

Fortunately, most of these end up as house dust (yep, really).

But there's a problem: Sometimes the cells lining the pores are not effectively shed. These excess cells plug pores, acting like a cork in a bottle. As a result, the sticky oil coming up from deep inside the pore can't escape. It accumulates and the *P. acnes* bacteria living inside the follicle go bananas because the oil is their food.

That's why the first step is to wash away as many excess dead skin cells as possible using a medicated exfoliating cleanser.

15

Give yourself
a hand.

As oil-gorging bacteria multiply behind closed pores, your body swings into action. The forces for good—your immune system's red and white blood cells—are sent in to fight what your body now senses is a raging infection. The collateral damage caused by the ensuing battle is redness, swelling and pus … and that's your pimple, zit, blemish.

A winning strategy against acne requires antibacterial weapons that are more proactive and precise than red or white blood cells—a more preemptive approach to reducing bacteria without inciting the inflammation.

A low-strength benzoyl peroxide lotion, applied to your whole face—and chest, back or shoulders, where needed—is an effective way to help your body fight acne bacteria *before* a battle begins.

16
Kills acne bacteria dead.

Benzoyl peroxide targets *P. acnes* like no other medicine.

It is antimicrobial, not antibiotic—the difference is technical but critical; it basically means the *P. acnes* bacteria cannot develop resistance to benzoyl peroxide's killing action. If the medicine works for you today, it will work for you tomorrow. The same can't be said for most oral antibiotics.

This is why benzoyl peroxide is the gold standard for fighting acne-causing bacteria.

A mild concentration of 2.5% is strong enough to be effective but gentle enough to use every day.

17
Benzoyl peroxide: clearer clears ... *and* whiter whites?

Benzoyl peroxide is a safe and trusted medicine, recommended by dermatologists for more than 40 years—with or without a prescription.

Found in the best-selling acne cleansers and lotions, benzoyl peroxide is an oxidizer (that's how it kills the nasty bacteria so efficiently).

When put inside your pores, benzoyl peroxide attacks and destroys *P. acnes* bacteria. When wiped on your towels, it bleaches color from fabrics.

It's easy to manage this routine once you're alert to the issue.

Use white towels. Don't pull a colored T-shirt over your head immediately after applying benzoyl peroxide medicines (get dressed before) and don't wipe excess on your jeans (yes, we know you do this).

18
Comedo is not funny.

What makes a blackhead black and a whitehead white? In both instances, we are talking about a hair follicle with a plugged opening—and each is called a "comedo."

The plug is dead skin cells, made sticky with oil. If this plug sits below the skin's surface, it's a whitehead; if the plug widens the pore and is exposed to air, it's a blackhead. (The darker color is not dirt; it's dead cells and oxidized oil when you get a good look at them.)

Left untreated, an unsightly comedo can nest comfortably in your skin for weeks or months, or erupt into a small-scale Mount Vesuvius.

Avoid pore-clogging makeup and moisturizers. Look for products labeled as "non-comedogenic," "non-acnegenic" or "oil-free" on either the product packaging or package insert.

19
Opening pores: the acid test.

"Acid" and "face" are two words most of us try not to use in the same sentence. However, there are a couple of acids that are just what the doctor ordered for breaking up plugged pores. One is glycolic acid, an excellent exfoliator—which means it removes excess dead skin cells.

The other is salicylic acid—"sal" acid to its friends—that helps to dissolve the plug itself.

They act like liquid pipe cleaners, and you'll find these active ingredients in cleansers, toners, leave-on lotions and masks.

This is why a toner is essential to your routine.

These acids won't work to clear your red bumps, but they do politely open the door for the other medicines that will.

20
Poor pores and follicle follies.

Your face has thousands of pores (about 10,000) that look like tiny holes dotting the skin's surface. We just want to say that pores look like tiny holes because they ARE tiny holes. The pore is the passageway leading from the top layer of your skin to the base of the hair follicle and oil gland. When everything is working right, the oil flows freely to the skin's surface—in appropriate amounts—helping keep it soft, supple, hydrated and healthy.

When not working right … well, you know what happens then.

Too much oil and a build-up of dead cells make pores bigger and cause blackheads and whiteheads.

Topicals containing glycolic, salicylic acid or retinol can help tighten them up. Smaller pores will look better and also be less prone to acne takeovers.

21

Not a lot of "foot-ne" out there. But everywhere else, watch out.

Wherever hair follicles and oil glands are in dense supply, acne finds a happy home.

The palms of your hands and soles of your feet are acne free because they are follicle free—but your face is dense with hair follicles, as are your chest, neck, shoulders, rear … and all are fair game for thriving acne bacteria.

Heat, moisture and friction bring out the best of bumps. Sitting in a warm office, driving for hours in your car, riding for miles on a mountain bike—all can trigger "back-ne" or "butt-ne."

When exercising, wear loose clothing and breathable fabrics; afterwards, shower as soon as you can—and use a medicated body wash. Treatments that work on your face work just as well anywhere else acne shows up.

22
The sensitive type.

A new skin-care product or topical medicine can sometimes bring out the red in you. And, reading the label or not, it's often hard to determine what ingredient is causing the trouble.

If you have concerns, apply (according to directions) a small amount to the soft, sensitive skin on your neck behind the ear lobe. Do this for three days; then wait.

No reaction: You're good to go!

A little red and dry: Proceed with caution and take on your new routine slowly, until your skin adjusts—maybe once a day or once every other day.

Itchy, red bumps or slight swelling: You've proved you're allergic to an ingredient in the product, so look for alternatives.

Know that your journey to clear skin should not be waylaid. Fewer than three percent of us have an allergy to benzoyl peroxide.

23
Too much of a good thing.

So here's something you probably didn't hear from your parents—it's possible to wash your face too often. In fact, if you have oily skin, you are probably overdoing it right now.

Your skin needs its natural oil to stay supple, hydrated and healthy … and you don't want to fight your skin.

So go easy on the soap.

Even if your acne-prone skin is dripping in oil, don't resort to using rubbing alcohol or frequent trips to the sink to clear it off. Over-cleansing and stripping tell your body, "Hey, my skin's surface is too dry so make more oil!" and it just gets worse from there.

A cleanser based on benzoyl peroxide is enough for most faces when used just twice a day.

24
Scrubs can be the pits.

There are earnest, well-meaning fans of facial scrubs that contain ground-up fruit parts—usually walnut or apricot pits—believing that such "natural" cleansing will deliver the deep-down clean that's bound to help clear up acne. Right?

Wrong.

The sharp edges from these particles actually causes micro-tears in your skin, leaving it raw and irritated—potentially making matters much worse.

You want to shed, not shred!

Small man-made polyethylene beads, which are smooth, round and uniform in size, provide just the right depth of exfoliation.

25
The irony of sulfur.

Sulfur, the biblical brimstone and one of the key ingredients of gunpowder, is also one of the oldest face-clearing medicines—an aid to putting out the fires of acne.

Yes, *that* sulfur.

Sulfur acts quickly and has many natural talents.

Sulfur masks are a great way to introduce this anti-acne ingredient into your routine. Some of the best use oil-absorbing kaolin clay in addition to sulfur to help reduce the redness and swelling that are the painful and visible flag bearers of acne.

Use a sulfur mask after a cleanser and before applying a toner, and don't be afraid to treat yourself two or three times a week.

26

With all those hair follicles, why don't I get "scalp-ne"?

You do get "scalp-ne"—it's called "dandruff."

Like coffee and cream or iced tea and lemon wedges, acne and dandruff are two that tango—especially among teenagers. Dandruff is triggered by the very same factors that fuel the acne cycle, with common yeast adding its own twist.

An oily, itchy, flaky scalp and pimply bumps will drive anyone crazy.

The treatment approach to dandruff is similar to that for acne—with medicines that reduce the shedding of skin cells or kill the yeast, or both. Topical cortisone also works.

While you are reading this, are your fingers searching for these annoying "scalp pimples?" If so, look for zinc pyrithione or salicylic acid as active ingredients in medicated shampoos.

27

Your skin is two-faced—and your face, two-skinned.

Just about everyone with acne has skin that is both oily and dry at the same time. Some areas are really oily, like the "T-zone" of your forehead, nose, upper cheeks and chin, while other areas are absolutely parched, like the sides of your face. This is because the density of oil-producing glands varies across the skin.

Your skin changes over time—and you can go from being a really oily-skinned teen to a really dry-skinned adult.

It might seem strange that dry skin can break out, but the acne-causing bacteria don't know or care about any of this. They are perfectly happy to keep the acne cycle going in any environment.

When it comes to acne, treat the process and then manage your skin type with an oil-free moisturizer for the dry parts or an oil-absorbing lotion for the shiny, oily regions.

28
Doctor your skin.

Sometimes you do everything right. You explore the full range of non-prescription acne treatments; you follow all the directions, take all the advice, think good thoughts.

But everyone's skin is unique. Some suffer more severe acne or are more prone to scarring.

If used properly from the start, the best over-the-counter medicines will work for the majority.

However, if your acne problem is not getting under control within six to eight weeks of starting your routine, please make an appointment to see a dermatologist—a physician dedicated to treating diseases of the skin.

Their arsenal includes antibiotics, retinoids, azelaic acid, sodium sulfacetamide—things you've never heard of but which have the potential to alleviate the most stubborn and severe cases. Gone are the days of endless oral antibiotics—we now have safe ways to heal and prevent acne.

29
Take a picture. You'll want to forget this.

Here's a step you'll want to skip, but please don't.

If you're reading this, acne has perhaps made your life a little smaller, a little sadder. But one day—really soon—acne will no longer have control over your life.

Honest.

And then you'll have "acne amnesia," because everyone wants to forget their bad skin.

Every once in a while, however, it's good to see where you came from—to measure how your commitment to new habits has paid off.

Your picture will remind you to never, ever go back to that place of helplessness.

So get a camera and snap one of those "before" photos. And if you ever share it with anyone, imagine the inspiration!

30

When it comes to beating acne, success is *routine*.

In one respect, acne is an ordinary skin condition—not life threatening and somewhat self-limiting.

But, in truth, acne is a profoundly serious disease—with a major impact on the quality of one's life, happiness and self-esteem.

There is a formula for getting acne out of your life that has proven its value on millions of faces—faces just like yours.

The key to your success will be staying committed—sticking to your medicated skin-care regimen day in and day out to *get* clear—and staying with your routine once you *are* clear.

Your acne didn't come up overnight, and it won't go away overnight. Be patient—clear skin will come.

You will succeed, and you will get back to feeling good again about that person you see in the mirror every morning.